"The Power of Womanhood

A Complete Guide to Women's Health"

ALEXIS SARRATT

Table of Content

Introduction 4

Chapter 1 5

Understanding your Body 5

Understanding the female Reproductive System's Anatomy and Physiology 5

Periodic Cycle 7

Hormone Adjustments..8

Chapter 2 10

Reproductive Health..10

Planning a Family and using Contraception....................13

Infertility and Conception 16

Conceiving and Giving Birth 19

Postnatal Wellness..22

Chapter 3 25

Sexual Health 25

Infections Transmitted Sexually (STIs)...........................27

A few Examples of STIs 28

Sexually Inappropriate 30

Good and Healthy Sexuality 33

Chapter 4 36

Psychological Health 36

Common Women's Mental Health Issues 38

Stress Reduction 41

Caring for Oneself and Mental Wellbeing 43

Chapter 5 46

Activity and Nutrition 46

Nutritional requirements and Healthy Eating practices 49

Physical Activity and Exercise for Women 51

Self-Esteem and Body Image 53

Chapter 6 56

Menopause and Aging 56

Premenstrual Syndrome and Menopause 58

Osteoporosis and Bone Wellness 61

Concerns about Age-related Health 63

Chapter 7 66

Healthcare and Advocacy 66

Getting Medical Care 69

Health Advocacy for Women 71

The Health of Women Worldwide 73

Conclusion 77

Introduction

Understanding and caring for your health as a woman is crucial to leading a successful life. A complicated and miraculous structure, the female body is capable of incredible feats of power and endurance. But, it is also susceptible to particular health issues and difficulties during a woman's life. An instruction manual called "The Power of Womanhood: A Complete Guide to Women's Health" aims to arm women with the information and abilities they need to take control of their health and wellness. This book offers helpful advice and resources for women of various ages and backgrounds on a wide range of topics, including nutrition, menopause, and reproductive health. "The Power of Womanhood" is the ideal travel companion on your path to optimum health and wellness, whether you are a young woman just beginning to explore your body and health or an older woman wanting to manage the changes and challenges of aging.

Chapter 1

Understanding your Body

To preserve excellent health and ward off potential health issues, women must understand their bodies and how they work. This chapter provides a thorough introduction to understanding your body, including topics like the menstrual cycle, hormonal changes, and the anatomy and physiology of the female reproductive system.

Understanding the female Reproductive System's Anatomy and Physiology

The female reproductive system is made up of internal and external organs that are in charge of egg creation, sperm fertilization, and the growth and nutrition of the fetus while a woman is pregnant.

The ovaries, fallopian tubes, uterus, and vagina are among the internal organs. On either side of the uterus, two tiny glands with an almond-like structure called the ovaries make and release eggs. Fertilization takes place in the fallopian tubes, two tiny tubes that connect the ovaries to the uterus. The fertilized egg can implant and develop during pregnancy in the uterus, a hollow, muscular organ. Sexual activity and childbirth take place in the muscular tube that connects the uterus to the exterior of the body, known as the vagina.

The vulva, clitoris, and labia are examples of external organs. The mons pubis, labia majora, labia minora, and clitoral hood are all parts of the vulva, which is the term for the external genital region. For sexual stimulation and pleasure, the clitoris—a tiny, extremely sensitive organ situated at the apex of the vulva—is crucial.

Knowing the anatomy and physiology of your body might make it easier for you to see potential health issues and get treatment when you need it.

Periodic Cycle

The monthly, normal menstrual cycle helps the female body get ready for pregnancy. Hormones generated by the pituitary, brain, and ovaries regulate it. The follicular phase, ovulatory phase, and luteal phase are the three phases that make up the menstrual cycle.

The follicular phase lasts roughly 14 days and starts on the first day of menstruation. The follicles in the ovaries start to mature and generate estrogen during this period, which gets the uterine lining ready for implantation.

At day 14 of the menstrual cycle, the mature follicle releases an egg into the fallopian tube, beginning the ovulatory phase. At this most fertile phase of the menstrual cycle, fertilization may take place if sperm are available.

After ovulation, the luteal phase starts and lasts for roughly 14 days. The empty follicle transforms into the corpus luteum during this stage and starts to release progesterone, which helps to thicken the uterine lining in preparation for implantation.

Hormone Adjustments

A woman experiences hormonal fluctuations throughout her life, which can significantly affect both her physical and mental well-being. The reproductive system benefits from the hormones progesterone and estrogen, which also help control the menstrual cycle.

Estrogen levels rise during puberty, which leads to the emergence of secondary sex traits such as pubic hair growth and breast development. Throughout the menstrual cycle, estrogen levels vary and fall during menopause, which can cause symptoms including hot flashes and vaginal dryness.

Progesterone levels change throughout the menstrual cycle as well and are important for maintaining pregnancy. Progesterone levels fall throughout menopause, which can cause symptoms like mood swings and insomnia.

Maintaining good health and avoiding potential health issues requires an understanding of your body. The anatomy and physiology of the female reproductive system, the menstrual cycle, and hormonal changes have all been thoroughly covered in this chapter. You can spot potential health issues and get medical assistance when necessary by getting to know your body.

Chapter 2

Reproductive Health

Emphasizes a key element of a woman's overall well-being. This section discusses a variety of reproductive health-related subjects, such as family planning and contraception, fertility and infertility, pregnancy and childbirth, and postpartum health.

This part describes several important reproductive health topics, including family planning and contraception. Women may find it difficult to select the best method given the wide range of contraceptive choices available. The various forms of contraception are thoroughly covered in this chapter, including hormonal techniques, barrier methods, and long-acting reversible contraceptives (LARCs), among others. It also emphasizes the value of family planning and provides instructions on how to decide when and how to start a family in an informed manner.

The section additionally addresses the subject of fertility and infertility, which for many women can be a cause of worry and emotional upheaval. It offers a thorough investigation of the variables that can impact fertility, such as age, dietary habits, and underlying medical issues. We also provide advice on how to improve your chances of getting pregnant, including tracking your ovulation, maintaining a healthy weight, and lowering your stress levels.

Although they can be incredibly joyful and transformative, pregnancy and childbirth also provide a unique set of difficulties. A plethora of knowledge on how to have a healthy pregnancy is provided in this chapter, including suggestions on prenatal care, diet, exercise, and self-care. It also discusses the stages of labor and delivery and provides advice on how to get ready for giving birth, such as by making a birth plan and taking pain treatment alternatives into account.

This section covers postpartum health, another crucial aspect of reproductive health. In particular, postpartum depression and anxiety are examined as well as other physical and psychological changes that women may go through in the days, weeks, and months following giving birth.

Also, it provides advice on how to look after oneself throughout this period, including healthy eating, exercise, and support from loved ones.

The Power of Womanhood: A Complete Guide to Women's Health Chapter 2 offers a thorough investigation of reproductive health, covering several subjects that are crucial for women to comprehend in taking charge of their health and well-being.

Planning a Family and using Contraception

Family planning and contraception are essential elements of reproductive health that empower women to make knowledgeable decisions about their bodies and lives. For women to be empowered and for gender equality to be achieved, they must have the freedom to decide when and if they want to have children.

Women can choose from a variety of contraceptive techniques, each of which has benefits and drawbacks. Birth control pills, patches, injections, and vaginal rings all use hormones to suppress ovulation and change the cervical mucus, which makes it more difficult for sperm to reach the egg. When applied correctly and consistently, these techniques are very successful, but they can also have negative side effects like nausea, migraines, and mood swings.

Condoms, diaphragms, and cervical caps, among other barrier methods of contraception, physically prevent sperm from reaching the egg. They are accessible for many women because they are freely available and do not need a prescription. They may also be less dependable than hormonal approaches and must be applied correctly every time to be effective.

IUDs and contraceptive implants are two examples of long-acting reversible contraception (LARC) treatments that are very effective and require less upkeep than other methods. Implants can last up to three years, and IUDs can last up to ten years. These procedures are risk-free and do not need daily monitoring, but they could have some unintended consequences, such as cramps or erratic bleeding.

To avoid having sex during your fertile window, charting your menstrual cycle is necessary for natural family planning. If used appropriately, this strategy can be quite beneficial, but it necessitates careful tracking and monitoring. For increased security, it can also be used in conjunction with other techniques.

The form of contraception that best fits each woman's unique needs, preferences, and medical history should be chosen. A healthcare professional's advice and support can be quite helpful while making these choices.

Beyond only using contraceptives, family planning also involves being able to schedule and plan pregnancies. This can lower the risk of unwanted births and enhance mother and child health outcomes. To advance women's empowerment and gender equality, it is crucial to increase access to family planning services, which is a human right.

For women to make educated decisions about their bodies and lives, contraception and family planning are critical elements of their reproductive health. We can help advance women's emancipation and raise people's health and welfare on a global scale by giving women access to a variety of tools and supporting their choices.

Infertility and Conception

Millions of people worldwide are impacted by the essential reproductive health issues of fertility and infertility. Infertility is the failure to conceive after one year of trying for women under the age of 35 or after six months for women over the age of 35. Fertility is the capacity to conceive and carry a pregnancy to term.

Infertility can be caused by a variety of reasons, including age, genetics, lifestyle choices, and underlying medical issues. Given that fertility decreases with age, especially beyond age 35, age is a key role. Fertility can also be impacted by lifestyle factors like stress, poor nutrition, smoking, drinking, and drug usage. Infertility can also be caused by medical diseases such as pelvic inflammatory disease (PID), endometriosis, and polycystic ovarian syndrome (PCOS).

Ovulation induction, intrauterine insemination (IUI), and in vitro fertilization are a few medical procedures that can help with fertility (IVF). By addressing underlying medical conditions or aiding in fertilization, these treatments seek to increase the likelihood of conception.

It is crucial to remember that infertility affects both men and women and that different causes may require different treatments. Infertility in men may be impacted by conditions including low sperm count, slow sperm motility, or erectile dysfunction. Medication, surgery, or assisted reproductive methods like intracytoplasmic sperm injection are all possible treatments (ICSI).

Along with medical interventions, lifestyle changes like better nutrition, lessened stress, and abstinence from alcohol and tobacco can also help increase fertility. For help managing the emotional and psychological effects of infertility, talking to a doctor or counselor might be beneficial.

It is crucial to remember that reproduction is a societal issue as well as a personal one. Promoting reproductive health and gender equality requires easy access to cost-effective fertility treatments and care. To improve reproductive results, it can be crucial to address the social and economic issues that cause infertility, such as poverty, a lack of education, and restricted access to healthcare.

Moreover, it should be noted that both fertility and infertility are significant components of reproductive health that have an impact on people and communities all over the world. Promoting reproductive health and gender equality requires an understanding of the causes of infertility as well as the available therapies and support alternatives. We can ensure that everyone has access to the care and support they require to fulfil their reproductive objectives by addressing the social, economic, and healthcare barriers to fertility care.

Conceiving and Giving Birth

One of the most life-altering events a woman may go through is pregnancy and childbirth. Pregnancy and labor are physically and emotionally demanding experiences that are loaded with joys and challenges from the moment of conception until the delivery of a healthy baby.

The growth and development of a fetus inside the womb is a complex process during pregnancy. A woman's body goes through a lot of changes during pregnancy to support the growing fetus, including hormone changes, weight gain, and modifications to the reproductive organs and systems.

To maintain the health of both the mother and the unborn child, women must receive appropriate prenatal care during their entire pregnancy. This involves visiting a doctor regularly, eating healthfully, exercising, and abstaining from dangerous substances like alcohol and tobacco.

The act of bringing a child out of the mother's womb is known as childbirth. Vaginal delivery, Cesarean section (C-section), and assisted vaginal delivery are some of the childbirth techniques available (e.g. with forceps or vacuum extraction).

Both the mother and the child may feel tremendous physical and mental pain during childbirth. The pain and discomfort of labor can be managed with the aid of pain-management measures, including prescription medication or organic methods like breathing exercises. The mother must have a strong birth team, which includes a medical professional and a birth partner, to support her emotionally and fight for what she needs during labor and delivery.

A woman's body goes through a lot of changes after giving birth as it heals and gets used to taking care of a kid. In addition to emotional changes like mood swings and adjusting to the duties of caring for a newborn, postpartum recovery can involve physical changes like bleeding, breast engorgement, and healing from any incisions or tears.

Breastfeeding is a crucial element of postpartum care because it helps the mother and baby form bonds and gives the newborn the nourishment and immune support it needs. But, breastfeeding can also be difficult and may call for assistance from lactation specialists or other medical professionals.

Overall, pregnancy and labor are challenging and life-changing processes that call for assistance, information, and appropriate medical care to protect both the mother's and the unborn child's health and well-being. Women can manage these events with greater assurance and comfort if they are aware of the psychological and physical changes that take place throughout pregnancy and childbirth and seek the appropriate prenatal and postpartum treatment.

Postnatal Wellness

An important component of a woman's overall well-being after childbirth is her postpartum health. A woman's body experiences multiple physical and hormonal changes while she heals and gets used to caring for a newborn infant after giving birth. Women should prioritize their postpartum health and get the attention they need to recover quickly.

Rest and healing are two of the most crucial components of postpartum wellness. The body requires time to recover from the physical stresses of labor and delivery after giving birth. This may entail getting enough rest and sleep, maintaining a balanced diet, drinking plenty of water, and avoiding physically demanding activities until a doctor has given the all-clear.

After giving birth, women may experience a variety of physical side effects, such as vaginal bleeding or discharge, perineal pain or discomfort, and breast engorgement or soreness. Along with weight increase or loss, stretch marks, and modifications to the breasts or abdomen, women may also suffer changes in their body size or form.

A crucial component of general well-being is postpartum mental health. After giving birth, many women go through a range of emotions, including happiness, excitement, and love for their newborn, as well as feelings of worry, melancholy, or overwhelm. These feelings are common and to be expected, but they can occasionally turn into postpartum. depression or anxiety, which can negatively affect a woman's mental health and general well-being

During the postpartum period, women must have the support and care they need for their mental health. This could entail speaking with a medical professional or mental health expert, joining a support group, or partaking in self-care practices like meditation or exercise.

Another crucial element of postpartum health for both the mother and the child is breastfeeding. Breast milk supports the baby's immune system and gives him or her vital nutrients, all while fostering emotional and bonding ties between mother and child. But, breastfeeding can also be difficult and may call for assistance and direction from lactation consultants or other medical professionals.

In general, a woman's postpartum health is a crucial component of her overall well-being. Women can manage the postpartum period more easily and confidently by prioritizing recovery and rest, getting help for their physical and emotional health, and practicing self-care.

Chapter 3

Sexual Health

Sexual health is the main topic of this chapter. Physical, emotional, and social well-being regarding sexuality are all key components of sexual health, which is a crucial component of overall well-being. This section discusses a variety of sexually health-related subjects, such as sexual anatomy and function, sexual pleasure, sexually transmitted diseases (STIs), and sexual consent.

Sexual anatomy and function are covered in Section 1. It examines the physiology of sexual arousal and response as well as the anatomy of the female reproductive system, including the external and internal genitalia. Also, it addresses common sexual issues like pain during sex, poor desire, and trouble eliciting orgasm while also offering solutions.

Section 2 discusses sexual gratification. It examines the various sexual pleasures, such as physical and emotional pleasure, as well as the importance of closeness and communication in sexual interactions. Also, it offers advice and techniques for heightening sexual gratification and investigating various modes of sexual expression.

STIs are covered in Section 3 of this chapter. It offers a general review of prevalent STIs, including information on their causes, symptoms, and available treatments. Also, it covers STD prevention techniques like safe sexual practices and routine STI testing.

Sexual consent is covered in Section 4. It examines the significance of permission in sexual experiences and offers advice on how to ask for and communicate consent. Additionally, it addresses widespread misconceptions regarding sexual consent and offers solutions for handling consent violations.

A complete review of sexual health is given in Chapter 3 of "The Power of Womanhood: A Comprehensive Guide to Women's Health," which is a crucial resource for women who want to give their sexual health top priority and navigate their sexual encounters with assurance and safety.

Infections Transmitted Sexually (STIs)

Infections known as sexually transmitted infections (STIs) are mainly spread through sexual contact. STIs come in a variety of forms and can affect anyone who engages in sexual activity. The various STI kinds, their signs and symptoms, and available treatments are covered in this section of "The Power of Womanhood: A Complete Reference to Women's Health."

A few Examples of STIs

Chlamydia: This bacterial infection can result in discharge, sex-related pain, and pelvic pain. Antibiotics can be used to treat it.

Similar to chlamydia in terms of symptoms, gonorrhea is a bacterial infection that, if left untreated, can result in more significant health issues. Antibiotics can also be used to treat it.

Herpes: is a viral illness that results in abrasive blisters or sores around the mouth or genital area. Antiviral medications can help manage outbreaks and lower the risk of transmission, even though there is no known treatment for herpes.

Genital warts: may develop as a result of the viral infection known as HPV, which is also connected to several cancers. Although there is no treatment for HPV, there is a vaccine that can guard against some viral strains.

HIV: is a virus that targets the immune system and, if left untreated, can result in AIDS. Antiretroviral therapy can help manage the illness and lower the risk of transmission, even though there is no known cure for HIV.

It's crucial to keep in mind that many STIs don't manifest any symptoms, making it possible for an infection to go undetected. Anyone who engages in sexual activity should regularly get tested for STIs because of this. A physical examination, blood tests, and/or vaginal swabs are all possible testing methods.

Utilizing condoms or dental dams during oral, vaginal, or anal sex is one way to prevent STIs. Additionally, it's critical to regularly get tested for STIs and to be open and honest with sexual partners about your status.

It's crucial to seek treatment as soon as possible if you are found to have an STI. Antibiotics and other drugs can be used to treat many STIs, and early diagnosis and treatment can help avert more serious health issues in the future. It's also crucial to tell any sexual partners so they can receive testing and care.

STIs can be a worrying topic, but learning about them and taking precautions can help lower the risk of infection and advance sexual health and well-being.

Sexually Inappropriate

The phrase "sexual dysfunction" is used to refer to a variety of problems that may make it difficult for someone to enjoy the sexual engagement. This can involve problems with arousal, discomfort, orgasm, or sexual desire. People of all ages and genders can experience sexual dysfunction, which can significantly influence their quality of life and general well-being.

Typical forms of Sexual Dysfunction

Low libido: This is the term for a lack of sexual desire that may be brought on by psychological or physical issues. Among them are hormone imbalances, drug interactions, depression, stress, and interpersonal connection problems.

A guy with erectile dysfunction is unable to obtain or sustain an erection during a sexual engagement. Physical conditions like diabetes or heart disease, as well as psychological conditions like sadness or anxiety, might contribute to this.

When a guy ejaculates too soon during sexual activity, frequently before they or their partner are pleased, this condition is known as premature ejaculation. Physical or psychological reasons may be to blame for this.

Vaginal dryness, infections, or diseases like endometriosis or pelvic inflammatory disease are just a few of the causes of painful intercourse.

Orgasm difficulty: This might be a physical or psychological problem that affects both men and women.

The underlying reason for sexual dysfunction will determine how it is treated. Some people may benefit from improved sexual function as a result of lifestyle modifications like exercise or stress management. For some disorders, doctors may also prescribe drugs like Viagra or hormone therapy. Psychological issues that can cause sexual dysfunction can also be addressed through counseling or therapy.

It's crucial to keep in mind that sexual dysfunction is a widespread problem, and getting help is nothing to be ashamed of. To properly diagnose and treat sexual dysfunction, an open conversation with sexual partners and healthcare professionals is essential. Many people with sexual dysfunction can enhance their sexual function and general quality of life with the proper support.

Good and Healthy Sexuality

A pleasant and respectful approach to sexual conduct and relationships that puts communication, safety, and mutual enjoyment first is referred to as "healthy sexuality." It's about having a sexual experience that is healthy, fulfilling, consenting, and respectful of everyone involved.

Communication: is a vital component of healthy sexuality. This entails being forthright and honest about your needs and goals with sexual partners, as well as establishing firm limits and respecting those of others. Before engaging in any sexual activity, it's crucial to obtain consent. You should also periodically check in with your partner(s) to make sure everyone is content and comfortable.

Another crucial component of healthy sexuality is engaging in safe sexual activity. This includes utilizing contraception to avoid an unexpected pregnancy as well as barrier measures like condoms or dental dams to guard against sexually transmitted illnesses. Maintaining sexual health also requires regular STI testing and an open conversation with sexual partners about their sexual health status.

A crucial component of good sexuality is self-care. This requires looking after your overall health—physically, mentally, and emotionally. This can involve doing things like maintaining good cleanliness, getting enough rest, eating a balanced diet, and working out frequently. It's crucial to prioritize your emotional and mental health by learning stress management techniques, developing self-compassion, and, if necessary, getting help from loved ones, friends, or mental health specialists.

It's crucial to remember that everyone's definition of healthy sexuality is unique, and no one solution works for everyone. You must experience sexual activity in a setting where you feel secure, respected, and in control. A healthy and respectful attitude toward sexuality can result in a fulfilling and enjoyable sexual life, regardless of whether you are in a committed relationship or are considering casual dating.

Chapter 4

Psychological Health

A vital component of total health and well-being is mental health. It refers to our psychological, emotional, and social health and can have a big impact on how we feel, act, and think. We will look at the value of mental health and how to preserve it in this chapter.

Taking care of our emotional and psychological needs is a necessary part of maintaining healthy mental health. This may consist of:

Taking the time to undertake activities that make you feel good, such as exercising, meditating, or spending time with loved ones, is referred to as practicing self-care.

When you are feeling overwhelmed or are having mental health problems, it's crucial to seek support from friends, family, or mental health specialists.

Handling stress: Stress is a natural part of life, but when it persists for an extended period, it may be harmful to our mental health. Using good coping mechanisms for stress, such as exercise, relaxation methods, or therapy, might lessen its effects.

Developing resilience: Our capacity to recover from challenging circumstances is referred to as resilience. Building resilience and enhancing mental health can be facilitated by cultivating coping mechanisms and a positive outlook.

Being aware includes being present at the moment and concentrating on the here and now rather than thinking about the past or the future. You can do this by meditating, doing deep breathing exercises, or just slowing down to enjoy the moment.

In addition to these methods, it's critical to recognize the warning signs and symptoms of mental health problems and to get assistance when necessary. Women frequently suffer from depression, anxiety, and eating problems as mental health issues. A mix of treatment, medicine, and lifestyle modifications can effectively address these problems, which can have a major negative influence on day-to-day life.

Prioritizing mental health as a critical component of general health and well-being is key. Women can enjoy happier, healthier, and more satisfying lives by taking steps to preserve excellent mental health and receiving assistance when necessary.

Common Women's Mental Health Issues

Women frequently experience mental health issues, which can negatively affect their quality of life. We examine typical mental health issues that women encounter and strategies for managing them in Chapter 4 of "The Power of Womanhood: A Complete Guide to Women's Health."

One of the most prevalent issues with women's mental health is depression. It may result in enduring melancholy, a sense of helplessness, and a loss of interest in once-pleasurable pursuits. Depression is more common in women than in men, and it can start for a variety of reasons, including hormonal changes, pregnancy, and menopause.

Medication, therapy, and lifestyle modifications like regular exercise and a balanced diet may all be part of the treatment for depression.

Another typical issue with women's mental health is anxiety disorders. Excessive concern, agitation, and trouble sleeping may be symptoms. Anxiety disorders are twice as common in women as in men, and they might start because of things like menopause, pregnancy, and hormonal changes. Therapy, medication, and lifestyle modifications like regular exercise, stress management, and relaxation techniques may all be used to treat anxiety disorders.

Anorexia and bulimia are two eating disorders that affect more women than men. These conditions may necessitate treatment in a specialized eating disorder treatment program because they can have a significant impact on both physical and mental health. Therapy, nutritional advice, and medication are all possible forms of treatment.

Some women have mental illness, a specific type of depression, after giving birth to a child. It might make it difficult to take care of oneself or one's child and can result in feelings of grief, anxiety, and weariness. Therapy, medicine, and assistance from family and friends may all be part of the treatment.

Women may also face other conditions like obsessive-compulsive disorder (OCD), post-traumatic stress disorder (PTSD), and borderline personality disorder (BPD) in addition to these prevalent mental health issues. Therapy, medication, and lifestyle modifications, including stress reduction and self-care, may all be used as part of the treatment for these illnesses.

Women ought to prioritize their mental health and seek assistance when necessary. Finding treatment can improve one's quality of life and general well-being. Mental health issues can have a big impact on daily living.

Stress Reduction

Many women feel stress frequently, which can have negative effects on their mental, emotional, and physical health. We'll look at ways to deal with stress so that women can improve their general well-being.

Many factors, such as those related to the job, family, relationships, finances, and health concerns, can cause stress. Unmanaged stress can result in both mental and emotional symptoms like anxiety and sadness as well as physical symptoms like headaches, stomach-aches, and muscle tension.

Using relaxation methods like deep breathing, meditation, and yoga is an efficient strategy to manage stress. These techniques can ease stress and foster a feeling of peace and well-being. Frequent exercise can help with mood and energy levels, which makes it an effective stress-management technique.

Self-care is a significant factor of stress management. This can entail partaking in enjoyable and unwinding pursuits like reading, taking a warm bath, or spending time with loved ones. It can also entail establishing limits and declining responsibilities that are putting too much strain on you.

Along with these methods, cognitive-behavioural therapy (CBT) can help people manage their stress. CBT entails working with a therapist to recognize and alter unfavourable thought processes and actions that increase stress.

It's crucial to keep in mind that stress management is a continuous process and that what works for one person may not work for another. It's crucial to try out various methods to determine which one suits you the best. It's crucial to seek medical assistance if stress is interfering with your daily life.

In addition, stress affects mental, emotional, and physical health and is a regular occurrence for women. Self-care, regular exercise, relaxation techniques, and cognitive-behavioural therapy are all excellent stress-reduction strategies.

To maintain a healthy and happy existence, it's crucial to prioritize stress management and get assistance when you need it.

Caring for Oneself and Mental Wellbeing

In today's fast-paced society, women frequently juggle multiple tasks and obligations, including raising children, managing careers, and upholding social relationships. In this section, we'll examine how self-care and mental wellness might support women in managing these demands while advancing their general health and well-being.

Self-care is the deliberate practice of attending to one's physical, emotional, and mental needs. Exercise, a nutritious diet, getting adequate sleep, and participating in hobbies or other fun activities can all contribute to this. Setting limits and declining demanding or stressful commitments are other examples.

Because self-care enables women to take time for themselves and recharge, it can have a good effect on mental wellness. Also, it can lessen the signs of anxiety and sadness and help avoid burnout.

In addition to self-care, obtaining expert assistance when necessary is a crucial component of mental wellness. Mental health specialists can offer assistance and direction in treating the symptoms of mental illness and creating coping mechanisms. In this situation, talk therapy, medicine, or a mix of the two may be used.

Additional methods for enhancing mental wellness include mindfulness and relaxation exercises like yoga, deep breathing, and meditation. These techniques can lessen tension and increase a feeling of peace and well-being.

It's crucial to keep in mind that maintaining mental well-being is a journey that calls for constant attention and care. To maintain a healthy and meaningful existence, women should put their needs first and seek assistance when necessary.

Women's health includes crucial facets such as self-care and emotional wellness. Self-care, getting help from a professional when necessary, and using relaxation techniques regularly can all support mental wellness and ward off burnout. Prioritizing mental health and taking care of oneself is crucial for leading a good and satisfying life.

Chapter 5

Activity and Nutrition

Examines the critical impact that diet and exercise play in preserving general health and fitness. Maintaining a healthy weight, lowering the risk of chronic diseases, and enhancing mental health all depend on a balanced diet and frequent exercise.

A healthy lifestyle includes proper nutrition as a major element. Women can maintain a healthy weight and lower their risk of developing chronic diseases like diabetes, heart disease, and certain types of cancer by eating a variety of healthy foods a variety of nutrient-dense foods including fruits, vegetables, whole grains, lean proteins, and healthy fats.

To prevent weight gain and health issues, it's crucial to pay attention to portion sizes and restrict the intake of processed and high-calorie foods. Furthermore important for maintaining hydration and enhancing general health is drinking plenty of water.

Another crucial element of a healthy lifestyle is exercise. Many health advantages of regular exercise include increased cardiovascular health, decreased chance of chronic diseases, and improved mental wellness.

Adults should engage in at least 150 minutes of moderate-intensity aerobic activity or 75 minutes of vigorous-intensity aerobic activity per week, as well as muscle-strengthening activities at least twice a week for a year, according to the Centers for Disease Control and Prevention (CDC).

Simple things like going for a brisk walk, riding your bike to work, or doing a fast workout at home can help you incorporate physical activity into your everyday life. Choosing a fun activity that fits into one's schedule will help to encourage sticking to a regular fitness plan.

In addition to diet and exercise, lifestyle elements like sleep and stress reduction significantly affect general health and wellness. Both physical and mental health depends on getting enough sleep, and stress management techniques can lower the chance of developing chronic illnesses and enhance mental health.

The Power of Womanhood: A Complete Guide to Women's Health's Chapter 5 places a strong emphasis on the value of good nutrition and regular exercise in leading a healthy lifestyle. Regular physical activity and a balanced diet full of nutrient-dense foods can lower the risk of chronic diseases and improve mental health. Setting other lifestyle priorities, such as getting enough sleep and managing stress, can also promote general health and wellness.

Nutritional requirements and Healthy Eating practices

Emphasizes the need of maintaining a balanced diet and getting the nutrition one requires. A healthy diet is crucial for general well-being and can help fend off chronic conditions like diabetes, heart disease, and obesity.

Consuming a range of nutrient-dense foods from all food groups is part of having healthy eating habits. This comprises fresh produce, entire grains, lean meats, and healthy fats. These foods give the body the vital vitamins, minerals, and fibber it requires to operate correctly.

Also, it's critical to pay attention to portion sizes and restrict the consumption of processed and calorie-dense foods. A balanced diet can lower the risk of chronic diseases and help women maintain a healthy weight.

Special dietary requirements apply to women, especially during pregnancy and breastfeeding. A woman's body needs more nutrients during pregnancy to support the fetus's growth and development. This entails consuming more calcium, iron, and folic acid. Also, some meals and drinks should be avoided by expectant mothers, including alcohol, unpasteurized dairy products, raw or undercooked meat, and seafood.

Breastfeeding mothers also have special nutritional demands, as breast milk delivers critical nutrients to the new-born. To stimulate milk production, breastfeeding women need extra calories and nutrients like calcium and vitamin D.

Also, women who are menopausal or postmenopausal may need to pay special attention to their nutritional needs. Women may need fewer calories as they become older, but more other nutrients, such as calcium and vitamin D, to maintain bone health.

A balanced diet rich in nutrient-dense foods can help prevent chronic diseases and maintain overall health. It's crucial to consider the specific nutritional requirements that women have at various phases of life to promote their overall health and well-being.

Physical Activity and Exercise for Women

Maintaining a healthy weight, enhancing cardiovascular health, and lowering the risk of chronic illnesses including type 2 diabetes, osteoporosis, and some types of cancer can all be achieved by women who engage in regular physical activity.

Furthermore beneficial to mental health, exercise can lower stress and lift the mood. Women who exercise frequently may feel more confident and have higher levels of self-worth.

Adults should perform at least 150 minutes of moderate-intensity aerobic activity or 75 minutes of vigorous-intensity aerobic activity each week, according to the Centers for Disease Control and Prevention (CDC). This translates into exercising for 30 minutes a day, five days a week.

To meet these objectives, women can pick from several physical activities, including walking, jogging, cycling, swimming, dancing, and strength training. For long-term adherence, it's critical to select pleasurable and viable activities.

Women should perform strength training exercises at least twice a week in addition to cardiovascular exercises. Strength training can enhance bone health, boost metabolism, and help you gain and retain muscle mass.

Pregnant or recently delivered women may require special considerations when exercising. Certain physical activities may need to be altered or avoided entirely when pregnant. Before the beginning or continuing a fitness regimen during pregnancy or postpartum, it's crucial to speak with a healthcare professional.

Emphasizes the value of physical activity and exercise for women. Frequent exercise has positive effects on both physical and mental health and can lower the risk of developing chronic diseases. In additament to strength training activities, women should strive for at least 150 minutes per week of moderate-intensity aerobic activity or 75 minutes

per week of vigorous-intensity aerobic activity. When beginning or continuing an exercise program during pregnancy or postpartum, it's vital to speak with a healthcare physician and to choose pleasurable and sustainable activities for long-term adherence.

Self-Esteem and Body Image

Self-esteem is a person's overall sense of worth and value, whereas body image is a person's opinion of their physical appearance.

Being unhappy with one's appearance can have a bad effect on one's general self-esteem, which is why body image and self-esteem can be strongly related. Women are frequently subjected to messages about the "perfect" body type, which causes them to have inflated expectations and unfavourable self-talk.

Low self-esteem and a negative body image can harm mental health, including depression and anxiety. To alter their appearance, women who deal with these difficulties might engage in hazardous habits like crash diets or excessive exercise.

When it comes to body image and self-esteem, women must place a high priority on self-care and self-acceptance. This can involve engaging in activities that bring joy and fulfilment, cultivating self-compassion, using positive self-talk, and surrounding oneself with encouraging individuals.

Physical exercise can make women feel confident and strong in their bodies, which can improve body image and self-esteem. Instead of only concentrating on how exercise and physical activity affects one's appearance, it's crucial to emphasize the benefits of these activities, such as how they make one feel.

In addition to self-care routines and exercise, women who struggle with poor body image and low self-esteem may find assistance from a mental health expert useful.

The relevance of body image and self-esteem for women's general health and well-being is emphasized in this chapter. Prioritizing self-care and self-acceptance is crucial since having a poor sense of one's body and low self-esteem can have a bad impact on mental health. Both engaging in physical activity and requesting help from a mental health expert can improve one's perception of one's physique and level of self-worth.

Chapter 6

Menopause and Aging

This chapter discusses menopause and aging. Women's bodies undergo major changes as they age, including a decline in estrogen production that triggers menopause. We'll offer advice and information on how women can control the physical and psychological changes brought on by aging and menopause.

Menopause, which signifies the completion of a woman's reproductive years, is one of the major themes discussed in this chapter. A natural biological process called menopause usually hits women in their 40s or 50s. Women may have a variety of symptoms during this time, such as mood swings, vaginal dryness, night sweats, and hot flashes.

We examine menopause symptom management approaches, such as hormone replacement therapy (HRT), which entails ingesting estrogen and progesterone to replenish the hormones that the body is no longer making naturally.

Other methods for treating menopause symptoms, including herbal supplements and lifestyle modifications, are also covered in this chapter.

The chapter addresses menopause as well as other health issues that may develop in older women, such as osteoporosis, which weakens and fractures bones, and cardiovascular disease, which is the primary killer of women.

This section offers suggestions on how women can maintain their health as they age, such as through consistent exercise, a nutritious diet, and frequent medical checks. It also emphasizes how crucial it is to maintain one's mental and emotional well-being, which can be done by doing things like spending time with loved ones and indulging in interests and hobbies.

We'll offer insightful advice on how women might handle the physical and psychological changes brought on by aging and menopause. Women can lead healthy, satisfying lives at any age by being aware of their bodies and taking proactive measures to maintain their health.

Premenstrual Syndrome and Menopause

A woman's physical and mental health may be significantly impacted by her perimenopause and menopause, two crucial life periods.

The transitional stage before menopause, known as perimenopause, can last anywhere from a few months to several years. Women's estrogen levels start to vary around this time, resulting in irregular periods and symptoms like hot flashes, mood swings, and sleep problems.

A woman is said to be in menopause when she has gone 12 months without a monthly cycle. Although it can happen earlier or later, this normally happens between the ages of 45 and 55. The end of a woman's reproductive years is marked by menopause, and the drop in estrogen levels can cause a range of symptoms, such as hot flashes, vaginal dryness, and mood swings.

Hormone replacement therapy (HRT), which involves taking estrogen and progesterone to replace the hormones that the body no longer produces, is one of the therapeutic options for controlling perimenopause and menopause symptoms that are covered in this chapter.

While HRT might help ease symptoms, it may also raise your risk of developing certain illnesses, like breast cancer and blood clots. Other methods for treating perimenopause and menopausal symptoms, including herbal supplements and lifestyle modifications, are also covered in this chapter.

Menopause and perimenopause can have a substantial impact on a woman's mental health in addition to the physical symptoms. We'll talk about the numerous emotional difficulties that women could have at this time, such as depression, mood swings, and worry. It also offers advice on how women can take control of their mental well-being, including methods like counseling, mindfulness exercises, and social support.

Overall, we'll offer helpful advice and information to help women negotiate the enormous changes brought on by perimenopause and menopause. Women can handle the symptoms and difficulties connected with these stages and lead healthy, full lives at any age by recognizing their bodies and taking proactive measures to maintain their physical and emotional health.

Osteoporosis and Bone Wellness

Women's bodies alter as they age in several ways that may have an impact on their bone health. The loss of bone density, which can result in osteoporosis, is one of the most important alterations. The condition osteoporosis weakens the bones, increasing their susceptibility to fractures and breaks.

Estrogen levels fall in women during menopause, and this hormone is crucial for maintaining bone health. Bone remodelling, or the process by which old bone is destroyed and new bone is produced, is regulated by estrogen. A drop in estrogen levels causes bone resorption (breakdown) to outpace bone creation, which lowers bone density.

Age, heredity, low body weight, smoking, heavy alcohol use, and some medications are just a few of the risk factors that might cause osteoporosis. Postmenopausal women, have a tiny physical frame, or have a family history of osteoporosis are more likely to acquire this illness.

Women should perform weight-bearing exercises like walking, jogging, and strength training to maintain strong bones and lower their chance of developing osteoporosis. These workouts aid in promoting bone density and bone growth. In addition, calcium and vitamin D, which are crucial elements for bone health, should be included in women's diets. Excellent sources of calcium and vitamin D are dairy products, leafy green vegetables, and fortified cereals.

Medication that can slow down bone loss or boost bone density may be helpful for women who are more likely to develop osteoporosis. One such medicine that can be used to treat osteoporosis is hormone treatment (HT). To maintain bone density and lower the risk of fractures, HT entails taking estrogen and progesterone supplements.

Women must consider bone health, especially as they get older. Women should be aware of their osteoporosis risk factors and take action to preserve strong bones through exercise, a good diet, and medication if required. Women can lower their risk of fractures and keep up an active, healthy lifestyle by putting bone health first.

Concerns about Age-related Health

Women may develop several gender-specific health issues as they get older. Others may be caused by hormonal changes that take place during menopause, while certain health problems may be inherited or the result of lifestyle decisions. Women should be aware of these potential health issues and take precautions to prevent and manage them.

Osteoporosis: is one of the most prevalent age-related health issues for women. Bones affected by this illness are weak and brittle, which increases the risk of breakage. Due to the drop in estrogen levels that occurs during menopause, women are more susceptible than males to developing osteoporosis. Women should engage in weight-bearing activity, consume a diet high in calcium and vitamin D, refrain from smoking, and limit their alcohol intake to lower their chance of getting osteoporosis.

Cardiovascular disease is another issue for women's health related to aging. Heart disease is a primary cause of death for both men and women, even though it is frequently considered a male health issue. Women may feel heart disease symptoms such as weariness, breathlessness, and nausea differently than males. Women should consume a diet low in saturated and trans fats, exercise regularly, and maintain a healthy weight to lower their chance of developing heart disease.

Another health issue that affects women more frequently as they age is breast cancer. While breast cancer can strike anyone at any age, the likelihood that a woman will get it rises with age. To identify any potential concerns early on, women should schedule routine mammograms and undertake regular self-examinations.

As women age, incontinence and problems with the pelvic floor may also become more prevalent. Several things, including childbirth, menopause, and obesity, might contribute to these disorders. By performing pelvic floor exercises and keeping a healthy weight, women can lower their risk of developing incontinence.

Women who are becoming older could also notice changes in their sexual health. Vaginal dryness and pain during sexual activity might be brought on by hormonal changes during menopause. Women may discuss options for controlling these symptoms with their healthcare physician, such as hormone replacement therapy or vaginal moisturizers.

Women should keep in mind that they can take charge of their health and welfare, even though aging can cause new health issues. Women can enjoy active, satisfying lives far into their golden years by keeping a healthy lifestyle and staying on top of preventive care.

Chapter 7

Healthcare and Advocacy

We'll talk about how crucial it is to support women's health and advocacy. All women have a fundamental right to access high-quality healthcare, so it's critical to understand your options. Also, a crucial component of enhancing healthcare for everyone is speaking up for your health as well as the health of others.

Healthcare access for women is hampered by prejudice, unequal access to care, and a lack of knowledge about preventive care. Being proactive in getting the treatment you require, such as routine checkups, preventive screenings, and managing chronic diseases, is crucial. An overview of some of the healthcare options for women will be given in this chapter, including insurance coverage, community health centers, and government initiatives.

To make sure that women receive the care they require, advocacy for women's health is also essential. This involves promoting laws that increase access to care, lessen inequalities and fund studies on women's health challenges. Participating in one of the numerous groups that promote women's health can significantly improve healthcare for all women.

Promoting health equity is a key component of healthcare advocacy. This entails tackling the underlying social and economic issues, such as poverty, racism, and discrimination, that cause health inequalities. Additionally, it entails making efforts to ensure that healthcare professionals are conscious of and attentive to the particular requirements of various communities, such as women of colour, women who identify as LGBTQ+, and women with disabilities.

It's critical to speak up for yourself and your loved ones in healthcare settings in addition to advocating at the policy level. This entails being an active participant in your care, seeking out second opinions, and asking questions. Assisting a friend or family member through a healthcare experience or assisting in educating others about their healthcare rights are two further examples of advocating for others.

Finally, this chapter will discuss how crucial it is for women to advocate for their mental health. Women have special difficulties getting access to mental healthcare, which is a crucial part of overall health. Several women's lives can be enhanced by advocating for mental health services and resources, lowering the stigma associated with mental illness, and encouraging mental well-being.

In general, advocacy and healthcare are essential to women's health. We can all fight to increase access to high-quality care and promote health equity for women everywhere by being aware, proactive, and engaged.

Getting Medical Care

Maintaining excellent health and wellness necessitates having access to healthcare. Sadly, many women encounter substantial obstacles when trying to receive healthcare, such as the scarcity of healthcare facilities in rural areas, a lack of health insurance, limited resources, and the stigma associated with specific health conditions.

Yet it's crucial to understand that every woman has a right to cheap, high-quality healthcare. Preventive care, such as routine checkups and screenings, as well as specialist care for particular medical conditions are included in this.

Developing a relationship with a primary care provider is among the best methods to get access to healthcare. A primary care provider is a medical expert who is in charge of organizing and supervising a patient's total medical care. When necessary, they can refer patients to experts, diagnose and treat ailments, and offer preventive care.

Numerous more healthcare specialists can offer specialized care for women in addition to primary care physicians. Gynecologists, obstetricians, midwives, mental health specialists, and dietitians are a few of these.

Health insurance is a crucial component of having access to healthcare. Preventive care, medical treatments, and prescription drugs are all covered by health insurance to some extent. In addition to government-funded programs like Medicaid and Medicare that offer healthcare coverage to qualified individuals, many firms provide health insurance as a reward to their workers.

It's also critical to understand that not everyone always has access to or can afford healthcare. Women who have healthcare difficulties might need to speak up for themselves and look for services to assist them in getting the care they need. Community health centers, no-cost or low-cost healthcare plans, and informational and supportive advocacy groups may fall under this category.

In general, women's health depends heavily on having access to healthcare. Women may take charge of their health and well-being and make sure they get the treatment they need by developing relationships with healthcare professionals, getting health insurance, and speaking up for themselves.

Health Advocacy for Women

Women's health advocacy is the practice of using a variety of tools to advance and defend the health and welfare of women. It entails raising awareness of women's health issues, fighting for laws and initiatives that support women's health, and giving women the tools they need to take charge of their health.

Eliminating inequities in women's healthcare access and outcomes is one of the key objectives of women's health advocacy. This includes making certain that women have access to inexpensive, all-inclusive healthcare services, such as preventative care, services related to reproductive health, and treatment for both acute and chronic illnesses.

The social and economic issues, such as poverty, discrimination, and violence, that have an impact on women's health are also addressed through advocacy initiatives. This involves speaking out in favour of laws promoting paid family leave, reasonably priced childcare, and equal pay as means of empowering women economically and socially.

The Health of Women Worldwide

Global women's health is a significant and complicated problem that includes a variety of health issues that have an impact on women all over the world. Women around the world confront particular health issues, such as access to resources, education, and healthcare, as well as cultural and societal norms that have an impact on their health outcomes.

Access to healthcare services is one of the main issues affecting the health of women worldwide. Many women in low-income nations lack access to fundamental healthcare services, such as family planning, maternal healthcare, and common sickness treatment. High rates of maternal mortality, STDs, and other health issues can result from this lack of access to healthcare, which can harm women's health.

The effects of poverty and economic inequality on women's health outcomes are a significant concern in the field of global women's health. Poor nutrition, a lack of access to sanitary facilities and clean water, and subpar housing are all factors that can have a detrimental effect on the health of women when poverty and economic disparity are present. In addition, gender-based violence, which may have a terrible effect on women's physical and emotional health, can be caused by poverty and economic inequality.

Global women's health is significantly influenced by cultural and social standards as well. Women may be reluctant to use healthcare services in some cultures because they are expected to put the needs of their families before their own. In addition, harmful practices like female genital mutilation, early marriage, and gender-based violence can be influenced by cultural and social norms, which can have detrimental effects on women's health.

Access to healthcare services must be improved, gender equality and women's empowerment must be promoted, and cultural and societal norms must be addressed to enhance the health of women worldwide. As part of this, organizations and clinics that assist women's health are given resources and support, and policies and initiatives that support women's health are advocated for.

Global women's health is a significant issue that calls for a multifaceted strategy to address the numerous difficulties that women face all over the world. We can make the world more just and equitable for all women by collaborating to promote women's health and provide women the tools they need to be in charge of their health outcomes.

Women's health advocacy also includes advancing research and innovation in this area and fighting for laws that ensure that women and different communities are fairly represented in clinical trials and research projects.

The promotion of women's rights and autonomy over their bodies and health decisions is a crucial component of women's health activism. In particular, this entails defending women's reproductive rights and promoting access to safe and legal abortion services.

In general, women's health advocacy is essential for improving women's health and well-being and making sure they have the tools and support they need to live happy, healthy lives.

Conclusion

A broad range of issues, including reproductive health, mental health, diet, exercise, aging and menopause, and healthcare activism, are covered in this comprehensive guide to women's health.

Women's health includes their mental, emotional, and social well-being in addition to their physical health. A woman's capacity to take charge of her health, make knowledgeable decisions about her body, and speak up for herself and other women is what gives women their power.

Women must be aware of their bodies' requirements for health, take action to prevent and manage health problems and ask for assistance when necessary. Women can live their best lives and reach their full potential in every area of life by taking care of their health.

It is also critical to recognize that not all women have equal access to resources and healthcare and that the health of women around the world continues to be a significant concern. Women all around the world struggle with several health issues, including discrimination, limited access to healthcare, and gender-based violence.

To guarantee that all women have access to the healthcare and resources they need to live healthy, meaningful lives, it is crucial to support and campaign for women's health on a worldwide basis.

In conclusion, this in-depth manual is a valuable tool for women of various ages and socioeconomic situations. Women may harness the power of womanhood to live healthy, happy, and full lives by taking charge of their health and standing up for both themselves and other women.

9 798389 916333